THE FOUR PHASE DIET

ELENA NICOLI

Copyright © 2019 Elena NICOLI

All rights reserved.

I BECOME WHAT I EAT.

I dedicate this book to all the people I have followed over the years in their physical and emotional changes.

CONTENTS

1	What you don't need to know	Pg 3
2	The principle of the four-phase diet	Pg 5
3	First week: hunger breaker plan spring-summer	Pg 9
4	First week: hunger breaker plan autumn-winter	Pg 16
5	Second week: detox plan spring-summer	Pg 23
6	Second week: detox plan autumn-winter	Pg 30
7	Third week: low glycemic index plan spring-summer	Pg 37
8	Third week: low glycemic index plan autumn-winter	Pg 44
9	Fourth week: Mixology spring-summer	Pg 51
10	Fourth week: Mixology autumn-winter	Pg 58

*Our body is a tool: we can use it to burden ourselves with matter
or to lift ourselves up to the divine*

1 WHAT YOU DON'T NEED TO KNOW

1. Raise your hand if you do not know the difference between a carbohydrate and a protein.

2. Raise your hand if you do not know that carbohydrates turn into sugars.

3. Raise your hand if you do not know the importance of introducing fiber into your diet.

4. Raise your hand if you do not know the advantages and disadvantages of a very long-term protein diet.

Those who raised their hands more than twice have surely run into the right book and can successfully continue reading and experimenting with this diet, for all the others (but I truly believe there are few of you) I advise you to research some basic notions on Google such as carbohydrates, proteins, fibers and vitamins so you too are ready to try the validity of the diet regime I have developed.

I am sure that after this premise you will be wondering if this book can really be the turning point you were looking for to improve your body by losing weight or if I am truly crazy and you are even more so for following me.
Well, even while distrusting those who define themselves as normal, I can assure that I have been working as a dietary biologist for many years and maybe it is the very practicality with which I like solving the problems of the people who turn to me that prompted me to write such a clear, easy, direct and effective book that respects what my clients usually ask me when they ask me for advice.

There are three reasons for which I find it unnecessary to lose and to make you lose time by listing very long notions of nutrition in this book and after you read them I am sure that you will agree with this choice.

-The first is that nearly every classic nutrition and diet book always has an introduction tied to the concepts listed above and if you have run into these books it is surely because you are curious to try a dietary approach that is new compared to the others you previously tried, therefore this is not the first diet book you have bought and you can surely find the basic notions of carbohydrates and proteins another way.

- Second: admitted but not granted that you read the notions of nutrition listed above I find that for purely practical purposes all that information is not of great use to you. It is one thing to know what a protein is but another knowing how to insert it correctly into a diet than can develop a specific organic response. Therefore, even if I explained to you all the details of proteins or any other type of food, it is not said that it is effectively clear to you how and where to correctly insert the foods by building a sensible diet plan. Therefore, it is better to let you see immediately how to manage foods in practice by following the dietary plans I have prepared.

- Third, I noted that most of the patients I saw in the surgery who have fought with their weight for years notionally speaking maybe know more than me (I am joking, however, I must say that the average person today is very well read on diets) but they have a problem with the application.

So, if I want to make my knowledge available to help improve the health of those who follow me I must be practical, easy and incisive and try to reach where any layman in nutritional science would never manage to make on his or her own, even after having read and documented the subject.

Therefore, let us cut the words and quickly get to the practice which is surely the aspect that interests you most.

2 THE PRINCIPLES OF THE FOUR PHSE DIET

I have called this the four phase diet for the very reason that I designed it thinking of the four weeks that make up a month and therefore this gives the chance to vary the food regime by offering four different modern dietary approaches that are integrated into a slimming process that, can be repeated over the year according to needs, or used in its cardinal principles as a healthy nutritional basis to be followed to keep in shape.

What will you experience over the next four weeks from a nutritional point of view?

1st WEEK: BREAKING THE HUNGER

Most people who diet generally come from a period in which excessive calories and recklessness with food ruled, usually with heavy consumption of major carbohydrates which created a dangerous vicious circle where carbohydrates called carbohydrates due to a metabolic logic linked to excessive secretion of insulin.

Therefore, the first step to come out of this impasse is to break this mechanism by putting the pancreas which was over stressed by the excessive carbohydrates of the previous months "at rest" for a week and so allow the body to start disposing some of the accumulated reserves.

In order to do this you must follow a mainly protein regimen that can drastically reduce the sense of hunger without causing any organic fatigue or harm to the body.

The regime that I will propose is deliberately proteic and not high protein where the latter term identifies instead a diet that is totally free of carbohydrates, including fruit which instead I included in any case, by nutritional choice, by evaluating and judging the daily glycemic charge which will deliberately be very low.

2nd WEEK DETOX

Having lowered the sense of hunger the time has come to drain the toxins from the body and so reduce the cellular inflammation that came from the abuse of calories in the previous months.

Paying attention to the acid-base balance of the body is very important for achieving good cellular response. In fact, it is well known how much animal proteins, sugars, alcohol or refined carbohydrates produce after having been eaten and metabolized, acidic wastes and how much the latter, if in excess, are able to create various organic disturbances known as tissue acidosis which is included as one of the symptoms.

- chronic tiredness/ drowsiness;
- irritability;
- muscular pain, concentration of lactic acid;
- joint pain, frequent inflammations;
- candidiasis, mycosis;
- frequent urinary tract infections;
- water retention, cellulite;
- osteoporosis;
- decalcification, demineralization.

Therefore, after having staunched the excessive need for food, it is important to start concentrating on raising the body's energy levels, with a diet that is rich in vitamins and antioxidants which are necessary for bringing the pH levels of the tissues back to basicity that is the parameter needed for activation of good cellular metabolic function.

3rd WEEK YES TO CARBHYDRATES BUT WITH LOW GLYCEMIC INDEX

You cannot live with only fruit extracts or only proteins, this is the reason that during this third week you will experience that the calculated use of well combined carbohydrates will never be the problem that can separate your body from weight loss.

I designed this plan in which I included low glycemic index carbohydrates, in other words, food with a high level of fiber or the specific combination with some proteins, that can avoid excessive secretion of insulin, the hormone that metabolically stimulates the presence of sugars but which we also know is the main anti-weight loss hormone if produced in excess.

You will experience at body level the difference in energy and the sense of being full you will develop by following the proposed combinations during the week compared to the simple wheat pasta garnished with some oil and parmesan, the classic dietary mistake made by most in the belief that eating a dietary meal, when instead the absence of vegetable fiber transforms the apparent and harmless wheat pasta into a super insulin bomb that can leave as its only effect the strong sense of after meal tiredness and after two or three fours a noticeable hunger for carbohydrates.

4th WEEK: MIXOLOGY

There is nothing better than mixing ingredients, this goes for life, in genetics and in the kitchen as it does in the approach to a diet.

Seven days in the name of a healthy diet, following the principles of the previous weeks so as to never get bored or tired, making the balancing game that is the basis of the dietary science increasingly varied.

APPLYING THE METHOD.
Here are some very important principles to read and follow carefully before starting:

- In the first week alcohol is completely forbidden, remember that wine and spirits are
liquid sugar and cannot be introduced in this phase. You can add in moderation two glasses of wine a week/or 2 beers in the following weeks (second, third and fourth).

- Completely eliminate the consumption of fizzy drinks.

- 2 cups of coffee per day are allowed, in the case you drink it with sugar we advise the use of Stevia as a sweetener.

- Cook the food with non-stick pans, using a little oil, a touch of salt and in the case of cooking vegetables add water to make them limp.

- Cook using only steam, grill or a non-stick pan, oven. Frying is banned.

- Let's not stress out by weighing grams of oil to garnish raw or cooked vegetables, we all know oil has a lot of calories and I sincerely think that nobody on a diet buys a precision balance to weigh 4-5 grams of oil on the tip of a spoon. Therefore the rule I ask you to follow for garnishing vegetables is to take the container of oil in the right hand, tilt it and pour a quick round of the circumference of the plate... I said quickly, if you do it slowly and at the end of the month you have not lost weight the fault is not mine as I warned you about making a quick round. Add a pinch of salt and vinegar (balsamic is good as well), or lemon if you have a slight lack of iron, the Vitamin C in the citrus will flavor the assimilation of non-heme iron, in other words of that iron contained in vegetables.

- Organize the time for the shopping and the subsequent preparation of the food, no excuse must stop you from preparing healthy lunches or dinners.
- Enjoy yourself by changing your habits, do not be too hard or strict with yourself. You are revolutionizing your way of eating and approaching a healthy diet. Every so often you will like what I offer, every so often you may turn up your nose, do not give up and enthusiastically live the new things you are experiencing.

- I have elaborated two variations for every week: on autumn-winter and one spring-summer, to give you the maximum chance to choose according to the time of the year in which you decide to begin the course.

- In some of the plans you will find some food in the following way: *bresaola* ... gram, which means the weight of the food you must look up in one of the tables that I placed at the end of the book, divided by weight of the person and gender (male or female)- .
If, for example you are a female who begins the path with a starting weight of 110 kg you must follow the grams of the food present in the column (female 120-90 kg) over the months, when you go down in weight and reach 85 kg you can change column (female 90-70 kg) and you will cook the meal according to the indicated weight.

- Unless specified otherwise the weight of the foods is understood as raw and free of scraps. It is important that you equip yourself with a normal kitchen food scale and that you do not cook the proposed portions by eye.

- I did not want to include some foods, such as pork and its derivatives (processed and cured ham, *mortadella*, salami) and salmon in the dietary plan for two simple reasons.

- Pork and especially its derivatives are highly inflammatory foods due to the presence of nitrates used for the preservation of the products and it is scientifically known that these substances can be transformed in the intestines into nitrosamines, potentially carcinogenic substances.

- While salmon is known for the levels of heavy metals it contains.
Now that I have explained everything you only have to follow the proposed plans and wait to see the results on your body.

3 FIRST WEEK:HUNGER BREAKER PLAN SPRING-SUMMER

MONDAY

BREAKFAST
Juice of 2 grapefruits + low-fat yogurt 250 g (you can also take it flavored with fruit) with 450 g of strawberries / or 2 cut peaches and 1 slice of melon (mix all together).

HALF MORNING
1 protein bar (found at the supermarket, of different brands, buy one that has at least 15% protein) +500 ml of water.

LUNCH
Chicken and pineapple salad: Chicken gr .... (see table) +1 slice of pineapple 1 cm thick. Cut the chicken into small cubes and, at the end of cooking, sauté it in a pan with the diced pineapple, add 100 gr of salad or rocket.

MIDDLE AFTERNOON
2 slices of melon / or 2 slices of pineapple 1 cm thick + 500 ml of water.

DINNER
Carpaccio of swordfish gr .... (see table; you find it in large hypermarkets) + at least 100 gr of raw vegetables to taste.

TUESDAY

BREAKFAST
400 ml of hot water with half a squeezed lemon + sheep or goat ricotta gr ... (see table) with corn cakes n:.... (see Table)

HALF MORNING
1 peach + 500 ml of water.

LUNCH
Cannellini bean salad: 1 jar of 240 gr cannellini beans (drained weight) with 100 g of salad or other raw vegetables to taste.

MIDDLE AFTERNOON
2 pink grapefruits + 500 ml of water.

DINNER
Cod or hake gr .... (see table) cooked in a pan with cherry tomatoes and capers + at least 100 gr of salad.

After dinner, wanting to drink an herbal tea to taste with a sprinkle of lemon, without sugar.

WEDNESDAY

BREAKFAST
Juice of 2 grapefruits + 250 g of soy yogurt flavored with vanilla with 200 g of raspberries / or 2 peaches

HALF MORNING
1 apple / or 500 grams of watermelon + 500 ml of water.

LUNCH
Tuna salad: 1 can of 125 g tuna + 100 g of raw vegetables to taste

MIDDLE AFTERNOON
1 protein bar (found at the supermarket, of different brands, buy one that has at least 15% protein) +500 ml of water.

DINNER
Avocado salad: 1 avocado + 100 g rocket + celery stalk + 1/2 fennel + half diced apple.

THURSDAY

BREAKFAST
400 ml of hot water with half a squeezed lemon + bresaola gr ... (see table) with corn cakes n:.... (see Table).

HALF MORNING
1 protein bar (found at the supermarket, of different brands, buy one that has at least 15% protein) +500 ml of water.

LUNCH
Roast beef gr .... (see food weight table) + at least 100 gr of raw vegetables to taste

MIDDLE AFTERNOON
2 slices of pineapple 1 cm / or 2 slices of melon + 500 ml of water.

DINNER
Eggs n .... (see table) with 3 small cubes of frozen spinach sautéed in the pan with the addition of a tablespoon of Parmesan cheese.

After dinner, wanting to drink an herbal tea to taste with a sprinkle of lemon, without sugar.

FRIDAY

BREAKFAST
Squeeze 2 grapefruits + low-fat yogurt 250 gr (you can also take it with fruit) with 2 tablespoons of flax seeds and 400 grams of strawberries / or 200 grams of raspberries.

HALF MORNING
1 protein bar (found at the supermarket, of different brands, buy one that has at least 15% protein) +500 ml of water.

LUNCH
Bresaola gr … (see table) + cherry tomatoes, rocket and some flakes of Parmesan cheese.

MIDDLE AFTERNOON
1 apple / or 500 grams of watermelon + 500 ml of water.

DINNER
1 medium-sized sea bream or sea bass baked with 1 grilled aubergine

After dinner, wanting to drink an herbal tea to taste with a sprinkle of lemon, without sugar

SATURDAY

BREAKFAST
Juice of 2 grapefruits + 2 whole fried eggs + 1 egg white with maize cakes n:…. (see Table).

HALF MORNING
1 protein bar (found at the supermarket, of different brands, buy one that has at least 15% protein) +500 ml of water.

LUNCH
Slice of tuna or grilled swordfish (see table) + at least 100 grams of raw vegetables to taste

MIDDLE AFTERNOON
2 peaches / or 1 apple + 500 ml of water.

DINNER
Free dinner (choose a second protein or meat to taste) + vegetable side dish (avoid potatoes in this phase and of course the bread)

After dinner, wanting to drink an herbal tea to taste with a sprinkle of lemon, without sugar.

SUNDAY

BREAKFAST
Squeeze 2 grapefruits + 250 gr of vanilla flavored soy yogurt with 2 slices of melon / or 400 grams of strawberries.

HALF MORNING
200 grams of raspberries + 500 ml of water.

LUNCH
1 vegetable burger to taste (of soy, legumes, vegetables; in this case women will eat only 1, while men if they felt very hungry can consume two) + at least 100 grams of raw vegetables to taste

MIDDLE AFTERNOON
500 grams of watermelon / or 1 apple + 500 ml of water.

DINNER
Chickpea hummus: in the mixer put 1 can of chickpeas (drained weight 240 g) + mint leaves, salt and oil to taste, half a squeezed lemon; blend all the ingredients together, if the mixture is too thick, add a dash of water and blend again + 1-2 raw fennel

4 FIRST WEEK: HUNGER BREAKER PLAN AUTUMN-WINTER

MONDAY

BREAKFAST
Juice of 2 grapefruits + low-fat yogurt 250 g (you can also take it flavored with fruit) with 2 tablespoons of pumpkin seeds and 1-2 kiwi cut into small pieces.

HALF MORNING
1 protein bar (found at the supermarket, of different brands, buy one that has at least 15% protein) +500 ml of water.

LUNCH
Chicken and broccoli salad: Chicken gr .... (see table) + 1-2 broccoli (you can also eat two large ones without affecting the final result). Cut the chicken into cubes and mix it with the broccoli, creating a single dish.

MIDDLE AFTERNOON
200 grams of fresh blueberries / or 2 slices of pineapple 1 cm thick + 500 ml of water.

DINNER
Lentils gr .... (see table) with tomato and celery + 100 gr of diced tofu (in this case the portion of tofu is the same for all) (single dish).

After dinner, wanting to drink an herbal tea to taste with a sprinkle of lemon, without sugar.

Insert chapter four text here. Insert chapter four text here. Insert chapter

TUESDAY

BREAKFAST
400 ml of hot water with half a squeezed lemon + sheep or goat ricotta or gr ... (see table) with corn cakes n:.... (see Table)

HALF MORNING
1 apple + 500 ml of water.

LUNCH
Bean soup with the addition of 40 grams of quinoa. If you are very hungry you can eat two full plates.

MIDDLE AFTERNOON
2 pink grapefruits + 500 ml of water.

DINNER
Cod or hake gr ... (see table) cooked in a pan with cherry tomatoes + at least 100 grams of salad.

After dinner, wanting to drink an herbal tea to taste with a sprinkle of lemon, without sugar.

WEDNESDAY

BREAKFAST
Squeeze 2 grapefruits + 250 gr of vanilla-flavored soy yogurt with 200 grams of fresh blueberries.

HALF MORNING
1 pear + 500 ml of water.

LUNCH
Tuna salad: 1 can of 125 g tuna + at least 100 g of raw vegetables to taste

MIDDLE AFTERNOON
3 mandarins / or 1 apple + 500 ml of water.

DINNER
Avocado salad: 1 avocado + 100 g rocket + celery stalk + 1/2 fennel + half diced apple.

After dinner, wanting to drink an herbal tea to taste with a sprinkle of lemon, without sugar.

THURSDAY

BREAKFAST
400 ml of hot water with half a squeezed lemon + bresaola gr ... (see table) with corn cakes n:.... (see Table).

HALF MORNING
1 protein bar (found at the supermarket, of different brands, buy one that has at least 15% protein) +500 ml of water.

LUNCH
Chickpea salad: 1 can of chickpeas of 240 grams (drained weight) with at least 100 grams of salad or other raw vegetables to taste.

MIDDLE AFTERNOON
2 slices of pineapple 1 cm thick + 500 ml of water.

DINNER
Eggs n .... (see table) with 3 small cubes of frozen spinach sautéed in the pan with the addition of a tablespoon of Parmesan cheese.

After dinner, wanting to drink an herbal tea to taste with a sprinkle of lemon, without sugar

FRIDAY

BREAKFAST
Juice of 2 grapefruits + low-fat yogurt 250 gr (you can also take it with fruit) with 2 tablespoons of flax seeds and 1 pear cut into small pieces.

HALF MORNING
1 protein bar (found at the supermarket, of different brands, buy one that has at least 15% protein) +500 ml of water.

LUNCH
Beef burgers gr ... (see table) + 1-2 cooked fennel / or 200 gr of cooked green bean

MIDDLE AFTERNOON
1-2 kiwis + 500 ml of water.

DINNER
1 medium-sized sea bream or sea bass made with 1 aubergine

After dinner, wanting to drink an herbal tea to taste with a sprinkle of lemon, without sugar.

SATURDAY

BREAKFAST
Juice of 2 grapefruits + 2 whole fried eggs + 1 egg white with corn cakes n:.... (see Table).

HALF MORNING
1 protein bar (found at the supermarket, of different brands, buy one that has at least 15% protein) +500 ml of water.

LUNCH
Slice of tuna or grilled swordfish (see table) +2 grilled zucchini.

MIDDLE AFTERNOON
3 mandarins / or 1 apple + 500 ml of water.

DINNER
Free dinner (choose a second protein or meat to taste) + vegetable side dish (avoid potatoes in this phase and of course the bread)

After dinner, wanting to drink an herbal tea to taste with a sprinkle of lemon, without sugar.

SUNDAY

BREAKFAST
Squeeze 2 grapefruits + 250 gr of vanilla-flavored soy yogurt with 200 grams of fresh blueberries.

HALF MORNING
1 pear + 500 ml of water.

LUNCH
1 vegetable burger to taste (of soy, legumes, vegetables; in this case women will eat only 1, while men if they felt very hungry can consume two) + at least 100 grams of raw vegetables to taste

MIDDLE AFTERNOON
3 mandarins / or 1 apple + 500 ml of water.

DINNER
Vegetable soup with the addition of 40 grams of quinoa. If you are very hungry you can eat two full plates

After dinner, wanting to drink an herbal tea to taste with a sprinkle of lemon, without sugar.

5 SECOND WEEK: DETOX PLAN SPRING-SUMMER

MONDAY

BREAKFAST
Juice of 2 grapefruits + low-fat yogurt 250 g (you can also take it flavored with fruit) with 450 g of strawberries / or 2 cut peaches and 1 slice of melon (mix all together).

HALF MORNING
600 grams of watermelon / or 2 slices of fresh pineapple + 500 ml of water.

LUNCH
Quinoa salad: Quinoa gr ... (see table) +2 zucchini. Sauté the zucchini in the pan and add the previously cooked quinoa (make a single dish)

MIDDLE AFTERNOON
2 slices of melon / or 2 slices of pineapple 1 cm thick + 500 ml of water.

DINNER
600-700 ml of fresh juice extract: 1 fennel+5 carrots+make volume with melon. If you feel that you could get very hungry, you can add 100 grams of raw vegetables to taste

TUESDAY

BREAKFAST
400 ml of hot water with half a squeezed lemon + corn noodles ... (see table) with a layer of jam without added sugar

HALF MORNING
3 apricots + 500 ml of water.

LUNCH
Cannellini bean salad: 1 can of 240 g cannellini beans (drained weight) with at least 100 g of salad or other raw vegetables to taste.

MIDDLE AFTERNOON
2 pink grapefruits + 500 ml of water.

DINNER
Mixed salad with feta: feta gr ... (see table) + cherry tomatoes + 1 tablespoon of capers + at least 100 g of rocket + corn cakes n ... (see table)

After dinner, wanting to drink an herbal tea to taste with a sprinkle of lemon, without sugar.

WEDNESDAY

BREAKFAST
Juice of 2 grapefruits + 400 grams of strawberries blended with 300 ml of vegetable milk (rice, oats, soy) / or 2 peaches and 1 slice of melon blended with 200 ml of vegetable milk

HALF MORNING
1 apple / or 500 grams of watermelon + 500 ml of water.

LUNCH
Fruit salad and yogurt: 200 grams of low-fat white yogurt + 2 slices of diced fresh pineapple + 150 grams of fresh raspberries + 1 diced banana

MIDDLE AFTERNOON
1 protein bar (found at the supermarket, of different brands, buy one that has at least 15% protein) +500 ml of water.

DINNER
Avocado salad: 1 avocado + 100 gr of rocket+ celery stalk + 1/2 fennel + half diced apple + corn cakes n .... (see table)

After dinner, wanting to drink an herbal tea to taste with a sprinkle of lemon, without sugar

THURSDAY

BREAKFAST
400 ml of hot water with half a lemon squeezed + 300 ml of water blended with 1 banana and 200 g of strawberries / or 1 banana and 200 g of blueberries / or 6 apricots.

HALF MORNING
500 ml of organic blueberry juice

LUNCH
Summer salad of tofu and pineapple: tofu gr .... (see food weight table) +1 stalk of celery + 100 gr of rocket or salad + 1 slice of pineapple cut into cubes + 8 almonds + biscuits n ... (see food weight table)

MIDDLE AFTERNOON
1 apple / or 2 slices of melon + 500 ml of water.

DINNER
600-700 ml of fresh juice extract: 300 g of watermelon + 2 peaches + make up to volume with melon. If you feel that you could get very hungry, you can add 100 grams of raw vegetables to taste

FRIDAY

BREAKFAST
Juice of 2 grapefruits + 350 ml of vegetable milk (rice, oats, spelled) + 3 handfuls of simple corn flakes.

HALF MORNING
1 protein bar (found at the supermarket, of different brands, buy one that has at least 15% protein) +500 ml of water.

LUNCH
Venus rice gr ... (see food weight table) + at least 200 grams of asparagus / or 2 courgettes (make a single dish)

MIDDLE AFTERNOON
1 apple / or 500 grams of watermelon + 500 ml of water.

DINNER
Coconut salad and vegetables: 4-5 diced coconut pieces + at least 80 grams of salad + 2 raw carrots + 1 celery stalk + 1 raw zucchini spaghetti (to make zucchini noodles or use a special tool called spiralizer, or it can be cut into thin strips using a mandolin) + corn cakes n ... (see table)

SATURDAY

BREAKFAST
500 ml of centrifuge: 1 fennel + 1 mango + 1 apple / or 2 peaches + make up to volume with carrots.

HALF MORNING
400 grams of cherries / or 1 apple + 500 ml of water.

LUNCH
Chickpea hummus: in the mixer put 1 can of chickpeas (drained weight 240 g) + mint leaves, salt and oil to taste, half a squeezed lemon; blend all the ingredients together, if the mixture is too thick, add a dash of water and blend again + at least 100 gr of raw vegetables to taste + corn cakes n ... (see table)

MIDDLE AFTERNOON
Organic blueberry juice with no added sugar 500 ml

DINNER
Free dinner (choose a second protein or meat to taste) + vegetable side dish (avoid potatoes in this phase and of course the bread)

SUNDAY

BREAKFAST
Squeeze 2 grapefruits + 250 gr of vanilla flavored soy yogurt with 2 slices of melon / or 400 grams of strawberries.

HALF MORNING
200 grams of raspberries + 500 ml of water.

LUNCH
1 vegetable burger to taste (of soy, legumes, vegetables; in this case women will eat only 1, while men if they felt very hungry can consume two) + at least 100 grams of raw vegetables to taste

MIDDLE AFTERNOON
500 grams of watermelon / or 1 apple + 500 ml of water.

DINNER
600-700 ml of fresh juice extract: 200 grams of raspberries + 3 slices of fresh pineapple + 2 slices of melon / or 1 apple + bring to volume with carrots or watermelon.

6 SECOND WEEK: DETOX PLAN AUTUMN-WINTER

MONDAY
BREAKFAST
4 orange juice + 2 bananas or 2 persimmons blended with 300 ml of vegetable milk.

HALF MORNING
500 ml of organic pomegranate juice with no added sugar

LUNCH
Venus rice gr ... (see table) with 1 broccoli

MIDDLE AFTERNOON
1 apple + 500 ml of water.

DINNER
600-700 ml of fresh juice extract: 1 fennel + 1 apple + 5 carrots + make volume with grapefruit. If you feel that you could get very hungry, you can add 100 grams of raw vegetables to taste

TUESDAY

BREAKFAST
400 ml of hot water with half a squeezed lemon + corn cakes n ... (see table) with a layer of jam without added sugar

HALF MORNING
200 grams of fresh blueberries + 500 ml of water.

LUNCH
Fennel and orange salad: 2 large finely cut fennels + 1-2 oranges cut into fine slices + 10 hazelnuts (chop the hazelnuts and sprinkle them over the vegetables) +corn cakes n ...... (see table)

MIDDLE AFTERNOON
2 pink grapefruits + 500 ml of water.

DINNER
Mixed vegetable soup (without the addition of pasta or rice; you can also eat two full dishes)

After dinner, wanting to drink an herbal tea to taste with a sprinkle of lemon, without sugar.

WEDNESDAY

BREAKFAST
Juice of 2 grapefruits + 1 banana + 2 kiwi blended with 300 ml of vegetable milk

HALF MORNING
1 apple / or 500 grams of watermelon + 500 ml of water.

LUNCH
Fruit salad and yogurt: 200 g of low-fat white yogurt + 5 almonds + 1 diced banana + 4 dates + 1 apple (mix everything together)

MIDDLE AFTERNOON
1 protein bar (found at the supermarket, of different brands, buy one that has at least 15% protein) +500 ml of water.

DINNER
Bean soup (without the addition of pasta or rice; you can also eat two full dishes).

After dinner, wanting to drink an herbal tea to taste with a sprinkle of lemon, without sugar.

THURSDAY

BREAKFAST
400 ml of hot water with half a squeezed lemon +corn cakes n ... (see table) with a layer of jam without added sugar.

HALF MORNING
1 apple + 500 ml of water.

LUNCH
Barley and mushroom salad: barley gr ... (see table) with 200 grams of champignon mushrooms. (Make a single dish)

MIDDLE AFTERNOON
1 apple / or 2 slices of melon + 500 ml of water.

DINNER
600-700 ml of fresh juice extract: 500 gr of fresh spinach + 2 apples + 3 kiwis + 1 fennel

FRIDAY

BREAKFAST
Juice of 2 grapefruits + 350 ml of vegetable milk (rice, oats, spelled) + 3 handfuls of simple corn flakes.

HALF MORNING
500 ml of organic pomegranate juice.

LUNCH
Venus rice gr ... (see food weight table) with 2 courgettes (make a single dish)

MIDDLE AFTERNOON
4 orange juice

DINNER
Cabbage salad: 100 g of cabbage + 1 diced apple + 5 walnuts + 1 stalk of celery + 1 tablespoon of dried red fruits +corn cakes n ... (see table)

After dinner, wanting to drink an herbal tea to taste with a sprinkle of lemon, without sugar.

SATURDAY

BREAKFAST
500 ml of centrifuge: 4 oranges + 1 pear + turmeric root + make up to volume with carrots.

HALF MORNING
400 grams of cherries / or 1 apple + 500 ml of water.

LUNCH
Corn pasta gr ... (see table) with 1 broccoli + at least 100 grams of raw vegetables to taste.

MIDDLE AFTERNOON
Organic blueberry juice with no added sugar 500 ml

DINNER
Free dinner (choose a second protein or meat to taste) + vegetable side dish (avoid potatoes in this phase and of course the bread)

After dinner, wanting to drink an herbal tea to taste with a sprinkle of lemon, without sugar.

SUNDAY

BREAKFAST
Squeeze 2 grapefruits + 250 gr of vanilla flavored soy yogurt with 1 banana and 1 diced pear + 1 sprinkle of cinnamon (mix all the ingredients together)

HALF MORNING
500 ml of organic pomegranate juice.

LUNCH
1 vegetable burger to taste (of soy, legumes, vegetables; in this case women will eat only 1, while men if they felt very hungry can consume two) + at least 100 grams of raw vegetables to taste

MIDDLE AFTERNOON
1 apple + 500 ml of water.

DINNER
600-700 ml of fresh juice extract: 1 pineapple + 3 oranges + ginger root + make up to volume with carrots

7 THIRD WEEK: LOW GLYCEMIC INDEX PLAN SPRING-SUMMER

MONDAY

BREAKFAST
Juice of 2 grapefruits + avocado mousse: 1 blended avocado with 250 ml of vanilla flavored soy milk + 2 tablespoons of bitter cocoa + 2 teaspoons of stevia.

HALF MORNING
1 protein bar (found at the supermarket, of different brands, buy one that has at least 15% protein) +500 ml of water.

LUNCH
Brown rice gr ... (see table) +1 courgette + 200 gr of already cooked borlotti beans. Make a single dish. Prepare a double portion to have lunch ready by Wednesday.

MIDDLE AFTERNOON
2 slices of melon / or 2 slices of pineapple 1 cm thick + 500 ml of water.

DINNER
Chicken salad: diced chicken breast gr ... (see table) + at least 100 grams of raw vegetables to taste +corn cakes n ... (see table)

TUESDAY

BREAKFAST
400 ml of hot water with half a squeezed lemon + sheep ricotta or goat gr ... (see table) with corn cakes n:.... (see Table)

HALF MORNING
1 peach + 500 ml of water.

LUNCH
Vegetable burger to taste (the quantity for women is 1 burger, while for men there are 2) + at least 100 g of raw vegetables to taste + corn cakes n:.... (see Table)

MIDDLE AFTERNOON
2 pink grapefruits + 500 ml of water.

DINNER
Quinoa salad: quinoa gr ... (see table) +6 olives + 1 courgette and an aubergine cut into cubes and stir-fried + basil (mix all the ingredients together)

After dinner, wanting to drink an herbal tea to taste with a sprinkle of lemon, without sugar.

WEDNESDAY

BREAKFAST
Juice of 2 grapefruits + 250 g of soy yogurt flavored with vanilla with 200 gr of raspberries / or 2 peaches

HALF MORNING
1 apple / or 500 grams of watermelon + 500 ml of water.

LUNCH
Brown rice gr ... (see table) +1 courgette + 180 gr of already cooked beans.

MIDDLE AFTERNOON
1 protein bar (found at the supermarket, of different brands, buy one that has at least 15% protein) +500 ml of water.

DINNER
Tuna salad: 1 can of 125 g tuna +100 g of raw vegetables to taste

After dinner, wanting to drink an herbal tea to taste with a sprinkle of lemon, without sugar.

THURSDAY

BREAKFAST
400 ml of hot water with half a lemon squeezed + 1 mango smoothie with 1 banana and 200 ml of vegetable milk

HALF MORNING
400 grams of strawberries / or 3 apricots + 500 ml of water.

LUNCH
Roast beef gr .... (see food weight table) +100 gr of raw vegetables to taste

MIDDLE AFTERNOON
2 slices of pineapple 1 cm / or 2 slices of melon + 500 ml of water.

DINNER
Eggs n .... (see table) with 3 small cubes of frozen spinach sautéed in the pan with the addition of a tablespoon of Parmesan cheese.

After dinner, wanting to drink an herbal tea to taste with a sprinkle of lemon, without sugar.

.

FRIDAY

BREAKFAST
Squeeze 2 grapefruits + low-fat yogurt 250 gr (you can also take it with fruit) with 2 tablespoons of flax seeds and 400 grams of strawberries / or 200 grams of raspberries.

HALF MORNING
1 protein bar (found at the supermarket, of different brands, buy one that has at least 15% protein) +500 ml of water.

LUNCH
1 sandwich of wholemeal bread about 80 g stuffed with 50 g of bresaola, spreadable thin cheese + rocket. Add 2 slices of pineapple as fruit at the end of this meal.

MIDDLE AFTERNOON
1 apple / or 500 grams of watermelon + 500 ml of water.

DINNER
Platter of tuna or grilled swordfish (see table) + at least 100 grams of raw vegetables to taste + corn cakes n:…. (see Table)

After dinner, wanting to drink an herbal tea to taste with a sprinkle of lemon, without sugar

SATURDAY

BREAKFAST
Juice of 2 grapefruits + corn cakes n ... (see table) with a layer of jam without added sugar.

HALF MORNING
1 low-fat yogurt + 500 ml of water.

LUNCH
Gr corn pasta (see table) with pesto + at least 100 gr of raw vegetables to taste. (Eating a plate of raw vegetables before or after the insertion of the paste, serves to keep the glycemic index of the pasta itself low and therefore a lower insulin response from the pancreas. If you want to stay in shape, never forget this very important step) .

MIDDLE AFTERNOON
2 peaches, or 3 apricots / or 1 apple + 500 ml of water.

DINNER
Free dinner (choose a second protein or meat to taste) + vegetable side dish (avoid potatoes in this phase and of course the bread)

After dinner, wanting to drink an herbal tea to taste with a sprinkle of lemon, without sugar

SUNDAY

BREAKFAST
Squeeze 2 grapefruits + 250 gr of vanilla flavored soy yogurt with 200 grams of raspberries / or 400 grams of strawberries.

HALF MORNING
2 slices of melon / or 1 apple + 500 ml of water.

LUNCH
Spelled pasta gr ... (see table) with tomato and mozzarella cubes +100 gr of raw vegetables to taste

MIDDLE AFTERNOON
500 grams of watermelon / or 1 apple + 500 ml of water.

DINNER
Chickpea hummus: in the mixer put 1 can of chickpeas (drained weight 240 g) + mint leaves, salt and oil to taste, half a squeezed lemon; blend all the ingredients together, if the mixture is too thick, add a dash of water and blend again + 1-2 raw fennel+ corn cakes n ... (see table)

After dinner, wanting to drink an herbal tea to taste with a sprinkle of lemon, without sugar.

8 THIRD WEEK:LOW GLYCEMIC INDEX PLAN AUTUMN-WINTER

MONDAY

BREAKFAST
Juice of 2 grapefruits + 2 bananas or 2 persimmons blended with 350 ml of vegetable milk.

HALF MORNING
1 protein bar (found at the supermarket, of different brands, buy one that has at least 15% protein) +500 ml of water.

LUNCH
Venus rice gr ... (see table) with 180 grams of lentils already cooked. (Tip: prepare a double portion to be kept in the fridge for lunch on Wednesday)

MIDDLE AFTERNOON
200 grams of fresh blueberries / or 2 slices of pineapple 1 cm thick + 500 ml of water.

DINNER
Hamburger gr ... (see table) +1 aubergine and 1 courgette baked +corn cake n ... (see table)

TUESDAY

BREAKFAST
400 ml of hot water with half a lemon squeezed + corn cakes n:.... (see table) with a veil of jam without added sugar.

HALF MORNING
1 pear + 500 ml of water.

LUNCH
Bean soup with the addition of 40 grams of quinoa. If you are very hungry you can eat two full plates.

MIDDLE AFTERNOON
2 pink grapefruits + 500 ml of water.

DINNER
Cod or hake gr .... (see table) cooked in a pan with cherry tomatoes +2 medium sized boiled potatoes.

After dinner, wanting to drink an herbal tea to taste with a sprinkle of lemon, without sugar.

WEDNESDAY

BREAKFAST
Squeeze 2 grapefruits + 250 gr of vanilla-flavored soy yogurt with 200 grams of fresh blueberries.

HALF MORNING
1 apple + 500 ml of water.

LUNCH
Venus rice gr ... (see table) with 180 grams of lentils already cooked.

MIDDLE AFTERNOON
3 mandarins / or 1 apple + 500 ml of water.

DINNER
Winter salad: 1 fennel + 1 sliced orange + radicchio + 8 walnuts + 1 stalk of celery +corn cakes n ... (see table)

After dinner, wanting to drink an herbal tea to taste with a sprinkle of lemon, without sugar.

THURSDAY

BREAKFAST
400 ml of hot water with half a squeezed lemon + 2 bananas or 2 persimmons blended with 350 ml of vegetable milk.

HALF MORNING
1 protein bar (found at the supermarket, of different brands, buy one that has at least 15% protein) +500 ml of water.

LUNCH
Cornmeal gr ... (see table) with ½ radicchio, 5 chopped walnuts and 2 tablespoons of Parmesan cheese +100 grams of raw vegetables to taste.

MIDDLE AFTERNOON
500 ml of organic pomegranate juice.

DINNER
Eggs n .... (see table) with 3 small cubes of frozen spinach sautéed in the pan with the addition of a tablespoon of Parmesan cheese.

After dinner, wanting to drink an herbal tea to taste with a sprinkle of lemon, without sugar.

FRIDAY

BREAKFAST
Juice of 2 grapefruits + low-fat yogurt 250 gr (you can also take it with fruit) with 2 tablespoons of flax seeds and 1 pear cut into small pieces.

HALF MORNING
1 protein bar (found at the supermarket, of different brands, buy one that has at least 15% protein) +500 ml of water.

LUNCH
Spelled gr ... (see table) with 1 large broccoli.

MIDDLE AFTERNOON
1-2 kiwis + 500 ml of water.

DINNER
1 medium-sized sea bream or sea bass cooked with vegetables to taste (cooked or raw)

After dinner, wanting to drink an herbal tea to taste with a sprinkle of lemon, without sugar.

SATURDAY

BREAKFAST
Juice of 2 grapefruits + oat porridge: 3-4 tablespoons of oat flakes cooked for some with some vegetable milk to obtain a thick cream without lumps + add 1 diced apple + cinnamon powder + 1 tbsp of maple syrup.

HALF MORNING
1 protein bar (found at the supermarket, of different brands, buy one that has at least 15% protein) +500 ml of water.

LUNCH
Basmati rice gr ... (see table) +3 tablespoons of cooked chickpeas (the canned ones are also fine) + 120 grams of chicken curry cubes.

MIDDLE AFTERNOON
3 mandarins / or 1 apple + 500 ml of water.

DINNER
Free dinner (choose a second protein or meat to taste) + vegetable side dish to taste

After dinner, wanting to drink an herbal tea to taste with a sprinkle of lemon, without sugar.

SUNDAY

BREAKFAST
Squeeze 2 grapefruits + 250 gr of vanilla-flavored soy yogurt with 200 grams of fresh blueberries.

HALF MORNING
1 pear + 500 ml of water.

LUNCH
Whole wheat pasta gr ... (see table) with 50 gr of green beans and 100 gr of diced Emmenthal cheese + at least 100 gr of raw vegetables to taste.

MIDDLE AFTERNOON
3 mandarins / or 1 apple + 500 ml of water.

DINNER
Chicken gr ... (see table) baked with baked vegetables: 1 carrot + half finely cut fennel + 1 courgette + 1/2 eggplant. Dust the vegetables with a little Parmesan cheese to create a crispy crust.

After dinner, wanting to drink an herbal tea to taste with a sprinkle of lemon, without sugar.

9 FORTH WEEK: MIXOLOGY SPRING-SUMMER

MONDAY

BREAKFAST
Juice of 2 grapefruits + low-fat yogurt 250 g (you can also take it flavored with fruit) with 450 g of strawberries / or 2 cut peaches and 1 slice of melon (mix all together).

HALF MORNING
1 protein bar (found at the supermarket, of different brands, buy one that has at least 15% protein) +500 ml of water.

LUNCH
Chicken and pineapple salad: Chicken gr .... (see table) +1 slice of pineapple 1 cm thick. Cut the chicken into small cubes and, towards the end of cooking, sauté it in a pan with the diced pineapple, add 100 gr of insalta or rocket.

MIDDLE AFTERNOON
2 slices of melon / or 2 slices of pineapple 1 cm thick + 500 ml of water.

DINNER
Carpaccio of sword gr .... (see table; you find it in large hypermarkets) +100 gr of raw vegetables to taste.

After dinner, wanting to drink an herbal tea to taste with a sprinkle of lemon, without sugar.

TUESDAY

BREAKFAST
Green tea 250 ml + low-fat yogurt 250 gr (you can also take it flavored with fruit) with 450 grams of strawberries / or 2 cut peaches and 1 slice of melon (mix all together).

HALF MORNING
600 grams of watermelon / or 2 slices of fresh pineapple + 500 ml of water.

LUNCH
Quinoa salad: Quinoa gr ... (see table) +2 zucchini. Sauté the zucchini in the pan and add the previously cooked quinoa (make a single dish)

MIDDLE AFTERNOON
2 slices of melon / or 2 slices of pineapple 1 cm thick + 500 ml of water.

DINNER
600-700 ml fresh juice extract: 1 fennel + 5 carrots + make volume with melon. If you feel that you could get very hungry, you can add 100 grams of raw vegetables to taste

WEDNESDAY

BREAKFAST
Squeeze 2 grapefruits + 200 grams of raspberries or 400 grams of strawberries + 1 banana blended with 300 ml of vegetable milk.

HALF MORNING
1 apple / or 500 grams of watermelon + 500 ml of water.

LUNCH
Brown rice gr ... (see table) +1 courgette + 200 gr of already cooked beans.

MIDDLE AFTERNOON
1 protein bar (found at the supermarket, of different brands, buy one that has at least 15% protein) +500 ml of water.

DINNER
Tuna salad: 1 can of 125 g tuna + at least 100 g of raw vegetables to taste

After dinner, wanting to drink an herbal tea to taste with a sprinkle of lemon, without sugar.

THURSDAY

BREAKFAST
400 ml of hot water with half a squeezed lemon + corn noodles ... (see table) with a layer of jam without added sugar

HALF MORNING
1 apple / or 500 grams of watermelon + 500 ml of water.

LUNCH
Fruit salad and yogurt: 200 grams of low-fat white yogurt + 2 slices of diced fresh pineapple + 150 grams of fresh raspberries + 1 diced banana

MIDDLE AFTERNOON
1 protein bar (found at the supermarket, of different brands, buy one that has at least 15% protein) +500 ml of water.

DINNER
Avocado salad: 1 avocado + 100 gr. Of rocket + celery stalk + 1/2 fennel + half diced apple +corn cakes n .... (see table)

After dinner, wanting to drink an herbal tea to taste with a sprinkle of lemon, without sugar.

FRIDAY

BREAKFAST
400 ml of hot water with half a squeezed lemon + bresaola gr ... (see table) with corn cakes n:.... (see Table).

HALF MORNING
1 protein bar (found at the supermarket, of different brands, buy one that has at least 15% protein) +500 ml of water.

LUNCH
Roast beef gr .... (see food weight table) +100 gr of raw vegetables to taste

MIDDLE AFTERNOON
2 slices of pineapple 1 cm / or 2 slices of melon + 500 ml of water.

DINNER
Eggs n .... (see table) with 3 small cubes of frozen spinach sautéed in the pan with the addition of a tablespoon of Parmesan cheese.

After dinner, wanting to drink an herbal tea to taste with a sprinkle of lemon, without sugar.

SATURDAY

BREAKFAST
Juice of 2 grapefruits + biscuits n ... (see table) with a layer of jam without added sugar.

HALF MORNING
500 ml of organic blueberry juice.

LUNCH
Gr corn pasta (see table) with pesto + at least 100 gr of raw vegetables to taste. (Eating a plate of raw vegetables before or after the insertion of the paste, serves to keep the glycemic index of the pasta itself low and therefore a lower insulin response from the pancreas. If you want to stay in shape, never forget this very important step) .

MIDDLE AFTERNOON
2 peaches, or 3 apricots / or 1 apple + 500 ml of water.

DINNER
Free dinner (choose a second protein or meat to taste) + vegetable side dish (avoid potatoes in this phase and of course the bread)

After dinner, wanting to drink an herbal tea to taste with a sprinkle of lemon, without sugar.

SUNDAY

BREAKFAST
Squeeze 2 grapefruits + 250 gr of vanilla flavored soy yogurt with 2 slices of melon / or 400 grams of strawberries.

HALF MORNING
200 grams of raspberries + 500 ml of water.

LUNCH
1 vegetable burger to taste (of soy, legumes, vegetables; in this case women will eat only 1, while men if they felt very hungry can consume two) + at least 100 grams of raw vegetables to taste

MIDDLE AFTERNOON
500 grams of watermelon / or 1 apple + 500 ml of water.

DINNER
600-700 ml of fresh juice extract: 400 grams of strawberries + 3 slices of fresh pineapple + make up to volume with pineapple / or 2 slices of melon + bring to volume with carrots or watermelon.

10 FOURTH WEEK: MIXOLOGY AUTUMN-WINTER

MONDAY

BREAKFAST
Juice of 2 grapefruits + low-fat yogurt 250 g (you can also take it flavored with fruit) with 2 tablespoons of pumpkin seeds and 1-2 kiwi cut into small pieces.

HALF MORNING
1 protein bar (found at the supermarket, of different brands, buy one that has at least 15% protein) +500 ml of water.

LUNCH
Chicken and broccoli salad: Chicken gr .... (see table) + 1-2 broccoli (you can also eat two large ones without affecting the final result). Cut the chicken into cubes and mix it with the broccoli, creating a single dish.

MIDDLE AFTERNOON
200 grams of fresh blueberries / or 2 slices of pineapple 1 cm thick + 500 ml of water.

DINNER
Lentils gr .... (see table) with tomato and celery + 100 gr of diced tofu (in this case the portion of tofu is the same for all) (single dish).

After dinner, wanting to drink an herbal tea to taste with a sprinkle of lemon, without sugar.

TUESDAY

BREAKFAST
4 orange juice + 2 bananas or 2 persimmons blended with 300 ml of vegetable milk.

HALF MORNING
500 ml of organic pomegranate juice with no added sugar

LUNCH
Venus rice gr ... (see table) with 1 broccoli

MIDDLE AFTERNOON
1 apple + 500 ml of water.

DINNER
600-700 ml of centrifuged: 1 fennel + 1 apple + 5 carrots + make volume with grapefruit. If you feel that you could get very hungry, you can add 100 grams of raw vegetables to taste

WEDNESDAY

BREAKFAST
400 ml of hot water with half a squeezed lemon + 2 bananas or 2 persimmons blended with 350 ml of vegetable milk.

HALF MORNING
1 protein bar (found at the supermarket, of different brands, buy one that has at least 15% protein) +500 ml of water.

LUNCH
Cornmeal gr ... (see table) with ½ radicchio, 5 chopped walnuts and 2 tablespoons of Parmesan cheese +100 grams of raw vegetables to taste.

MIDDLE AFTERNOON
500 ml of organic pomegranate juice.

DINNER
Eggs n .... (see table) with 3 small cubes of frozen spinach sautéed in the pan with the addition of a tablespoon of Parmesan cheese.

After dinner, wanting to drink an herbal tea to taste with a sprinkle of lemon, without sugar.

THURSDAY

BREAKFAST
Juice of 2 grapefruits + low-fat yogurt 250 gr (you can also take it with fruit) with 2 tablespoons of flax seeds and 1 pear cut into small pieces.

HALF MORNING
1 protein bar (found at the supermarket, of different brands, buy one that has at least 15% protein) +500 ml of water.

LUNCH
Beef burgers gr ... (see table) + 1-2 cooked fennel / or 200 gr of cooked green beans

MIDDLE AFTERNOON
1-2 kiwis + 500 ml of water.

DINNER
1 medium-sized sea bream or sea bass made with 1 aubergine

After dinner, wanting to drink an herbal tea to taste with a sprinkle of lemon, without sugar

FRIDAY

BREAKFAST
Squeeze 2 grapefruits + 250 gr of vanilla-flavored soy yogurt with 200 grams of fresh blueberries.

HALF MORNING
1 apple + 500 ml of water.

LUNCH
Venus rice gr ... (see table) with 180 grams of lentils already cooked.

MIDDLE AFTERNOON
3 mandarins / or 1 apple + 500 ml of water.

DINNER
Winter salad: 1 fennel + 1 sliced orange + radicchio + 5 walnuts + 1 stalk of celery + corn cake n ... (see table)

After dinner, wanting to drink an herbal tea to taste with a sprinkle of lemon, without sugar.

SATURDAY

BREAKFAST

Juice of 2 grapefruits + biscuits n ... (see table) with a layer of jam without added sugar.

HALF MORNING
500 ml of organic pomegranate juice with no added sugar

LUNCH
Corn pasta gr... (see table) with pesto + at least 100 gr of raw vegetables to taste. (Eating a plate of raw vegetables before or after the insertion of the paste, serves to keep the glycemic index of the pasta itself low and therefore a lower insulin response from the pancreas. If you want to stay in shape, never forget this very important step) .

MIDDLE AFTERNOON
2 peaches, or 3 apricots / or 1 apple + 500 ml of water.

DINNER
Free dinner (choose a second protein or meat to taste) + vegetable side dish (avoid potatoes in this phase and of course the bread)

SUNDAY

BREAKFAST
Squeeze 2 grapefruits + 250 gr of vanilla-flavored soy yogurt with 200 grams of fresh blueberries.

HALF MORNING
1 apple + 500 ml of water.

LUNCH
Venus rice gr ... (see table) with 180 grams of lentils already cooked.

MIDDLE AFTERNOON
500 ml grape centrifuge.

DINNER
Winter salad: 1 primosale cheese + 1 fennel + 1 sliced orange + radicchio + 1 stalk of celery +corn cake n ... (see table)

TABLE WOMAN: WEIGHT PERSON > 120 KG/ FOOD gr

- Bresaola 110 gr
- Carpaccio of sword 150 gr
- Spelled / barley (cereal) 100 gr
- Feta cheese 150 gr
- Corn cakes 4 biscuits
- Beef burger 200 gr
- Cooked lentils 240 gr
- Raw lentils 120 gr
- Cod / hake 250 gr
- Whole wheat pasta 100 gr
- Spelled corn pasta 120 gr
- Chicken 220 gr
- Quinoa 120 gr
- Ricotta cheese 150 gr
- Brown rice and venus 120 gr
- Roast beef 130 gr
- Tuna / sword steak 200 gr
- Eggs 3

TABLE WOMAN: WEIGHT PERSON 120-90 KG/ FOOD gr
- Bresaola 100 gr
- Carpaccio of sword 130 gr
- Spelled / barley (cereal) 90 gr
- Feta cheese 130 gr
- Corn cakes 3 biscuits
- Beef burger 180 gr
- Cooked lentils 220 gr
- Raw lentils 110 gr
- Cod / hake 220 gr
- Whole wheat pasta 100 gr
- Spelled corn pasta 100-110 gr
- Chicken 200 gr
- Quinoa 100 gr
- Ricotta cheese 140 gr
- Brown rice and venus 100 gr
- Roast beef 120 gr
- Tuna / sword steak 180 gr
- Eggs 3

TABLE WOMAN: WEIGHT PERSON 90-70 KG/ FOOD gr
- Bresaola 80 gr
- Carpaccio of sword 100 gr
- Spelled / barley (cereal) 80 gr
- Feta cheese 120 gr
- Corn cakes 3 biscuits
- Beef burger 180-160 gr
- Cooked lentils 200 gr
- Raw lentils 100 gr
- Cod / hake 180 gr
- Whole wheat pasta 90 gr
- Spelled/corn pasta 90-100 gr
- Chicken 180 gr
- Quinoa 90 gr
- Ricotta cheese 120 gr
- Brown rice and venus 90 gr
- Roast beef 100 gr
- Tuna / sword steak 160 gr
- Eggs 2

TABLE WOMAN: WEIGHT PERSON 70-50 KG/ FOOD gr
- Bresaola 70 gr
- Carpaccio of sword 80 gr
- Spelled / barley (cereal) 70 gr
- Feta cheese 100 gr
- Corn cakes 2 biscuits
- Beef burger 150 gr
- Cooked lentils 200-180 gr
- Raw lentils 90 gr
- Cod / hake 160 gr
- Whole wheat pasta 80 gr
- Spelled/corn pasta 80 gr
- Chicken 160 gr
- Quinoa 80 gr
- Ricotta cheese 100 gr
- Brown rice and venus 80 gr
- Roast beef 90-80 gr
- Tuna / sword steak 150 gr
- Eggs 2

TABLE MAN: WEIGHT PERSON > 140 KG/ FOOD gr

- Bresaola 140 gr
- Carpaccio of sword 180 gr
- Spelled / barley (cereal) 130 gr
- Feta cheese 170 gr
- Corn cakes 5 biscuits
- Beef burger 220 gr
- Cooked lentils 270 gr
- Raw lentils 130 gr
- Cod / hake 280 gr
- Whole wheat pasta 130 gr
- Spelled/corn pasta 150 gr
- Chicken 250 gr
- Quinoa 140 gr
- Ricotta cheese 170 gr
- Brown rice and venus 150 gr
- Roast beef 150 gr
- Tuna / sword steak 250 gr
- Eggs 4

TABLE MAN: WEIGHT PERSON 140-120 KG/ FOOD gr

- Bresaola 130 gr
- Carpaccio of sword 150 gr
- Spelled / barley (cereal) 120 gr
- Feta cheese 150 gr
- Corn cakes 4 biscuits
- Beef burger 220 gr
- Cooked lentils 250 gr
- Raw lentils 120 gr
- Cod / hake 250 gr
- Whole wheat pasta 120 gr
- Spelled/corn pasta 130 gr
- Chicken 230 gr
- Quinoa 130 gr
- Ricotta cheese 160 gr
- Brown rice and venus 130 gr
- Roast beef 130 gr
- Tuna / sword steak 230 gr
- Eggs 4

TABLE MAN: WEIGHT PERSON 120-90 KG/ FOOD gr

THE FOUR PHASE DIET

- Bresaola 120 gr
- Carpaccio of sword 120 gr
- Spelled / barley (cereal) 110 gr
- Feta cheese 130 gr
- Corn cakes 3 biscuits
- Beef burger 200 gr
- Cooked lentils 230 gr
- Raw lentils 110 gr
- Cod / hake 230 gr
- Whole wheat pasta 100 gr
- Spelled/corn pasta 120 gr
- Chicken 200 gr
- Quinoa 120 gr
- Ricotta cheese 150 gr
- Brown rice and venus 120 gr
- Roast beef 120 gr
- Tuna / sword steak 200 gr
- Eggs 3

TABLE MAN: WEIGHT PERSON 90-80 KG/ FOOD gr

- Bresaola 90-100 gr
- Carpaccio of sword 100 gr
- Spelled / barley (cereal) 10-90 gr
- Feta cheese 130 gr
- Corn cakes 2-3 biscuits
- Beef burger 180 gr
- Cooked lentils 200 gr
- Raw lentils 100 gr
- Cod / hake 200 gr
- Whole wheat pasta 100 gr
- Spelled/corn pasta 110 gr
- Chicken 180 gr
- Quinoa 110-100 gr
- Ricotta cheese 140 gr
- Brown rice and venus 110-100 gr
- Roast beef 110 gr
- Tuna / sword steak 180 gr
- Eggs 3

NOW IT IS UP TO YOU

I am sure that you have carefully followed the diet, even if with some mistakes on the rules, at the end of the month your body would have lost a certain number of kilos.

Now that you have achieved this good result what will you do?

Certainly not go back to the previous habits. In fact, I remind you that the meaning of the word diet is not tied to restriction or privation but a healthy life style and therefore try to treasure this month, maybe by repeating the dietary plan during the year and by enjoying yourself by making some healthy changes to my proposals.

Nutritional and dietary science are basically an art, and the art of learning the subtle game of balancing what to give yourself and what to give up, I give myself a culinary extra by knowing that I will then have to give my body some (two or three) days of food control in order to allow the excretory organs to dispose of and rebalance the "damage" caused by the dinner with friends, by the birthday, the celebration and the extended aperitif. ...

However, we all know that the complex problem of weight often hides traces of an emotional malaise that finds in food a companion for temporary and fragile gratification.

We eat in excess due to dissatisfaction, anger, disappointment, loneliness, anxiety, betrayal or for any other uncontrolled emotion that is however capable of directing the system towards the chasm of insecurity and insatiable anxiety.

Over the years the strong impact of these situations on a satisfactory dietary result led me to develop a method of rebalancing nutrition that takes into consideration all these aspects and created a holistic approach to the traditional dietary guidelines that can integrate body-emotions-mind and soul.

I call this method Nutrimentum in which feeding the soul and the body knowingly is the central focus of my work. I accompany people in real paths of self awareness through food and helping to overcome emotional blockages that keep them imprisoned in a body that they feel does not belong to them and does not reflect their being. In order to reach all this I bring together various knowledge and sciences: biochemistry, psychosomatics, flower therapy, phytotherapy, kinesiology and yoga.

For further information you can visit my website: www.nutrimentum.net

I hope that with this step you have taken will be the first towards a long-lasting path of inner change that I am certain will accompany you for the rest of your life with curiosity.

ABOUT THE AUTHOR

I'm a Biologist specialized in human nutrition and psychosomatic disorder.
Hatha yoga teacher
I lead people through paths of nutritional awareness and personal growth.

Printed in Great Britain
by Amazon